Reversing Diabetes

The Herbal Medicine Approach

Joanna Aphiah

Reversing Diabetes: The Herbal Medicine Approach by Joanna Aphiah.

Published by Kwizbud Publishing House, 204C Chestnut Crossing Dr.,Newark 19713, New Jersey, U.S.A.

Books@kwizbud.com

Copyright © **2019 Joanna Aphiah**

ISBN: 9781097892747

Table of Contents

PREFACE

Reversing Diabetes: The Herbal Medicine Approach is a book written as a daily companion for diabetics, or their friends and relatives.

All I know about herbs and testimonies from people with diabetes who have successfully reversed their diabetes and now living free of their doctor's medication are all carefully recorded.

Reversing diabetes refers to that state in which the patient's insulin needs are minimal and some persons having diabetes may discover that they can maintain healthy or almost normal blood sugar level requiring little or no insulin. If you diligently adhere to the recommendations and herbal recipes in this book, before long, you should be giving your testimony also.

Tremendous research has gone into this book to ensure it comes out as a one-in-all handbook on causes, herbal treatment, and reversal of diabetes.

3 John 1: 2 "Beloved I wish above all things that thou mayest prosper and be in health, even as thy soul prospereth.

Joanna Aphiah

iv

Attaining remarkable health is not difficult. The human body knows how to stay healthy. All we have to do is give our body outstanding nutrition then it has the building materials it requires to heal disease and restore itself from the inside out. You must also avoid all of the food ingredients and foods that cause disease.

More than 95% of all chronic disease today, is caused by food choice, lack of physical exercise, toxic food ingredients, and nutritional deficiencies.

–Mike Adams

Facts on Diabetes

The United States Dept of Health & Human Services, Centers for Disease Control and Prevention (CDC) reliably informs that more than 30 million Americans are living with diabetes, representing a ratio of 1 sufferer in every 10 Americans. And CDC further posits that 90% to 95% of the identified population have type 2 diabetes. Type 2 diabetes is most prevalent in people over age forty-five, though it is not uncommon to find it in children, teens, and young adults also. Obesity rates in children are rising, just like rates of type 2 diabetes in youth. And it has been observed that over 75% of children with type 2 diabetes have a family member who has it, too. But this identified relationship is not always genetic or because the persons are related; it could be because certain habits are common to both individuals by proximity.

It would be keen to note that many people have type 2 diabetes without knowing it because the symptoms don't make you feel unwell. United Kingdom's National Health Service (NHS) says you're more at risk of developing type 2 diabetes if you are:

i)   over 40 years of age (or 25 years for South Asian persons)

ii)   have a close relative (such as a parent, brother or sister)previously diagnosed with diabetes

iii)   you are overweight or obese and lastly

iv)   you are of South Asian, Chinese, African Caribbean or black African origin by ancestral heritage, not a place of birth citizenship.

The hormone insulin is made in the pancreas, and it triggers the cells in your body to convert blood sugar into energy. If a person has type 2 diabetes, his cells do not respond to insulin, referred to as insulin resistance, resulting in your pancreas producing more insulin in an attempt to make the cells to react accordingly. Due to your cell resistance, your blood sugar rises even while your insulin level is very high. High blood sugar damages the body and can cause other serious health problems, such as vision loss, kidney disease, and heart disease.

First symptoms of type 1 diabetes appear as soon as blood sugar hits high levels. Symptoms include fatigue, hunger, thirst, blurred vision, weight loss, tingling or numbness in the feet, and frequent urination. Extremely high blood sugar can cause rapid breathing, nausea, fruity breath, and dry skin.

On the other hand, symptoms of type 2 diabetes don't start as early as symptoms of type 1 diabetes. For many years, the first symptoms of type 2 diabetes may not show up — meaning diabetes may have caused irreparable damage to a person's body without them realizing it. For this reason, type 2 diabetes could be dubbed as the worst type of diabetes. First symptoms include fatigue, frequent urination, thirst, pain or numbness in the hands or feet hunger, blurred vision, recurrent infections, and erectile dysfunction in men.

Noticeable symptoms for type 2 diabetes include but is not limited to the following:

i)   blurred vision

ii)   feeling very tired with little or no physical activity

iii)   frequent peeing, particularly at night

iv)   feeling thirsty all the time

v)   losing weight without intention

vi)   wounds or cuts taking longer to heal

vii)   itching around your vagina or penis, or repeatedly getting thrush

So if you have noticed any of the symptoms above you need to visit your doctor. Though some of the symptoms may be indicative of other diseases and not related to diabetes, however, in many cases, most people tend to overlook or not understand these symptoms even when they have been there for some time as they may associate it to something else due to lack of awareness. So most often, people with diabetes are identified for the first time when they go to the hospital for blood or urine tests for something else, only to be informed by the doctor that high level of sugar was found in their blood setting the stage for prediabetes and type 2 diabetes.

Generally, the doctor will go on to talk to you about:

i.   what diabetes is

ii.   What high blood sugar means for your health

iii. What medication you'll have to take

iv.   your diet and exercise

v.   your lifestyle – for example, alcohol and smoking

Why you are Reading this Book

You are reading this book because you have diabetes or you have a close relative who has it. It is also likely that you are reading this book to stay informed or for preventive purposes. Diabetes is a very deadly disease. It is a killer and at the very least complications (Alzheimer's disease, Foot damage, Kidney damage (nephropathy), Nerve damage (neuropathy), Eye damage (retinopathy), Skin conditions, Hearing impairment, Cardiovascular disease) resulting from diabetes is irreversible and devastating. My knowledge of this fact increases the burden on me not only to provide you with enough or complete information but rather to give information that may be few in wording but yet very useful in solving the problem. That said, it is equally apt to note that my responsibility as a herbal medicine practitioner ends in providing you with tested herbal remedies. The remedies have been known to work without side-effects for ages while it is your greater responsibility to take action in implementing the solutions provided in this book and staying faithful to your treatment program even though the maintenance program to avoid a recurrence.

If you are not already practicing meditation and fasting combined for a powerful healing medium, then you are not only missing out but also living in risk. Risk of sudden illness or death. I will urge you to read my book "Meditation and Fasting Combined: A Powerful Healer." The book will help you build the discipline required to tap into your spiritual healing powers. Where medications don't work, meditation and fasting surely do. It comes in different formats. You can get the Kindle format for less than a dollar.

To make "Reversing Diabetes: The Herbal Medicine Approach" a complete guide, I have answered and provided evidence to most of the frequently asked questions by people living with diabetes. Comments and opinions from recovering diabetics are also included because they have a therapeutic effect equivalent to over a thousand medicines. The morale booster of seeing or hearing from someone who has overcome what you are still struggling with is infectious and quite enormous.

Reversing diabetes is an expression that usually refers to a considerable long-term enhancement in insulin sensitivity in persons with type 2 diabetes. With dedication and time, type 2 diabetes can be reversed, and the outcome can be very gratifying, with less tiredness and better holistic health. Persons with type 2 diabetes that can get their HgA1C below 42 mmol/mol (6%) without taking diabetes medication are said to have resolved or reversed their diabetes. This is also referred to as putting diabetes into remission.

For a person living with diabetes, Loss of body weight is beneficial in helping to reverse the progression of diabetes.

Diabetes is not a death sentence; it's just a medical term that means too much sugar in your blood. After all, they had to call it something. Simply put, we don't eat as they did 100 years ago when people often only had one meal a day. Most of the diabetes is formed by overeating and eating at the wrong time extended over time coupled with minimal exercise if any. No thanks to our mostly sedentary modern lifestyle; from our mattress beds to comfy sofas then our cars and ergonomic office chairs, the cycle continues till we are so obese. Example: many people eat breakfast, then snack, eat lunch, then snack, eat dinner, then a snack before bed. Add on the beers, juices, energy drinks;

milkshakes, ice creams and soft drinks that are always present in these snacks, then you will understand how much our eating culture and lifestyle have nosedived. As such, most people overeat for no reason at all, and that is the most common reason for diabetes. The other is what you eat, and the most popular snack is ice cream, cookies, cakes, and so on.

If you think you have come to the point where you can discontinue your diabetes medication, ensure you speak to your doctor or physician before doing so.

Testing and Diagnosing Types of Diabetes

Persons having type 1 diabetes do not produce adequate insulin, and as a result, sugar accumulates in their blood instead of being absorbed into the cells, where it is required as a hormone for regulating blood sugar. In type 1 diabetes, high blood sugar causes symptoms like hunger, fatigue, and thirst. Type1 diabetes can cause terrible consequences, including damage to the blood vessels, nerves, and other internal organs. Some related complications of type1 diabetes apply in type 2 also. The difference is that persons with type 2 diabetes produce enough insulin; but their body cells pose resistance to utilizing the insulin resulting in the pancreas producing more and yet more insulin, which is what causes the complications of both excess blood sugar as well as excess insulin in the body that causes obesity.

3.1 Getting Tested:

To determine if you have prediabetes, type 1, type 2, gestational diabetes or otherwise, you'll have to test your blood sugar. As such your doctor will request you perform at least one of the under-listed tests to ascertain your condition:

A1C Test

This test estimates your average blood sugar level over two to three months. An A1C under 5.7% is ok, while from 5.7 to 6.4% indicates you have prediabetes, and higher than 6.5% indicates you have diabetes.

Fasting Blood Sugar Test

Accurately estimate your blood sugar after an overnight fast. A fasting blood sugar level lower than 99 mg/dL is desirable, 100 to 125 mg/dL shows you have prediabetes, and 126 mg/dL or above indicates you have diabetes.

Glucose Tolerance Test

Will measure your blood sugar levels before and after you drink some glucose. This test also requires you'll fast overnight before having your blood drawn to determine your fasting blood sugar level. So this test is usually done just after the Fasting blood sugar test. Next, you drink the glucose solution and have your blood sugar level checked one (1) hour, two (2) hours, and if possible three (3) hours afterward. At 2 hours, a blood sugar level lower than 140 mg/dL is considered acceptable, 140 to 199 mg/dL shows you have prediabetes, and 200 mg/dL or higher means you have diabetes.

Random Blood Sugar Test

This checks your blood sugar at the time you are being tested irrespective of whether you have eaten or not. You can perform this test at any time and don't need to fast first. A blood sugar level of 200 mg/dL or higher indicates you have diabetes.

3.2 Diagnosing Type1 or Type2 or Gestational Diabetes:

Blood Test For Autoantibodies

If your doctor thinks you have type 1 diabetes, your blood should also be examined for the presence of autoantibodies. This test quickly isolates the particular type between type 1 and type 2 because autoantibodies are absent in type 2 diabetes but present in type 1 diabetes. Autoantibodies are substances that indicate your body is attacking itself.

Urine Test For Ketones

Your urine should be tested for ketones (produced when your body burns fat for energy), which if present, indicates type 1 diabetes or type 2 diabetes when absent in the urine.

Blood Test For Gestational Diabetes

Higher than acceptable Blood sugar, early in pregnancy, may indicate you have type 2 or type 1 diabetes rather than gestational diabetes. Gestational diabetes is diagnosed using blood tests and should be carried out between 24 and 28 weeks of pregnancy. If you possess more risk factors for having gestational diabetes, then your doctor may request your test earlier.

Disease Status	TEST			
	A1C	Fasting Blood Sugar	Random Blood Sugar	Glucose Tolerance
Diabetes	6.5% or above	126 mg/dL or above	200 mg/dL or above	200 mg/dL or above
PreDiabetes	5.7 – 6.4%	100 – 125 mg/dL	N/A	140 – 199 mg/dL
Normal	Below 5.7%	99 mg/dL or below	N/A	140 mg/dL or below

Source: American Diabetes Association

3.3 Regular Maintenance Test

You need to check your blood sugar regularly. Ask your doctor how frequently you should test it and what your expected blood sugar levels should be. Maintaining your blood sugar levels as close to the target as possible will help you prevent or delay diabetes-related complications.

People with types 1 and 2 diabetes need to check their blood sugar level with a device called a glucometer about four times a day to know their sugar levels.

The A1C test is a blood sugar test that gives information about your average levels of blood sugar, also called blood glucose, over three months. The A1C check can be used to diagnose prediabetes and type 2 diabetes. The A1C test is also the primary test used for diabetes management.

Most Accurate Test For Diabetes:

A fasting blood glucose level from 100 to 125 mg/dL (5.6 to 6.9 mmol/L) means the person has prediabetes. If it's higher than 126 mg/dL (7 mmol/L) on two separate tests, it implies diabetes has been identified. Oral glucose tolerance test. This test requires that you fast overnight, and the fasting blood sugar level is measured.

Dangerous Level of Diabetes:

If your blood sugar level is above 600 milligrams per deciliter (mg/dL), or 33.3 millimoles per liter (mmol/L), this condition is referred to as a diabetic hyperosmolar syndrome. Safe blood sugar level For the average person is 70 to 105 mg/dl in a fasting state. Safe blood sugar level is the optimum range that safely provides the body with adequate amounts of energy.

Severely high blood sugar turns your blood thick and syrupy. Diabetes is identified when the fasting blood sugar level is at or above 126 mg/dl.

3.4 Testing Your Diabetes Meter:

It is recommended that you test any meter you intend to use at home for regular checks before commencement of use. To verify the meter do the following: Check your blood sugar level with your meter at the same time that you are drawing blood for a laboratory test. Compare the lab test result with your meter result. If your meter Results are within 15 percent of the lab result, then your meter is good and suitable for your regular home testing. These meters are often referred to as "interstitial glucose measuring devices."

You prick your finger with a sharp needle, apply a drop of blood on a test strip, and then place the strip into the meter that shows your blood sugar levels. Meters vary in cost, portability, readability, speed, size, and features such as larger displays or spoken instructions for those with impaired vision. Most meters deliver results in less than 15 seconds and store this information for later use.

Some meters also compute an average blood sugar level over a specified time. Some devices incorporate software kits that display graphs and charts of your past test results.

Some devices let you test your upper arm, forearm, thigh, and the base of the thumb.

These results could differ from the blood sugar levels gotten from a fingertip stick.

Levels in the fingertips display changes faster. This is quite useful during a test when your blood sugar is rapidly changing, like after exercise or after a meal.

Also if you have symptoms of low blood sugar, the fingertip stick test is the best, don't trust test results from other parts of your body.

Some devices come combined with insulin pumps; however, they're not as reliable as fingertip stick glucose results.

Testimonies of Diabetics

Dennis Pollock of the Spirit of Grace ministries has made significant contributions to understanding the treatment of diabetes, by interviewing people with diabetes. Pollock talks about Kenneth Woolard, who has reversed his diabetes. His blood sugar was very high; it went above the range of the blood sugar device he was using (which reads up to 500). Ken was flirting with a disability and early death, but he found the salvation he needed and got his blood sugar levels down - drastically down that his A1c levels now indicate that not only is Ken no longer diabetic, but he is, in fact, healthy.

I have included comments by many sufferers here because it is best learning from other peoples experience. A person with diabetes has something very unique to learn from another person with diabetes that even the most acclaimed physician in the world can't teach. So bring out your paper and pen and get ready to learn from diabetics all over the world. However, note that I am in no way endorsing the recommendation or opinions contained in any of the testimonies below.

Most of the comments and opinions in the testimonies below have been adequately addressed in various sections of this book with my views and the results of many research investigations discussed.

Jeff C

You are what you eat. If you eat garbage, your body will be garbage. It's as easy as that.

The biggest problem is people take things on faith (faith is belief without evidence). This has brought us all to a place where many are eating super processed food full of refined carbs and sugar using an utterly wrong food guide. Educate yourselves.

Philly J.

I found that I can eat a banana and it doesn't raise my sugar too high; I can even eat two times a day. Right now I eat one but only before I exercise, and I do hard work for two and a half hours. If I don't eat carbs at all, I see myself ready to faint in the gymnasium, so I eat some banana before I workout and only on training days. I also use "blood glucose" by Nature's, and it works better than metformin. I can state that the low carb diet is working to help lower my A1C. I use apple, cider vinegar as well and along with the herbs and no grains or sweets, I don't have to take medication for my diabetes.

Kyle M

You are over exaggerating by saying 190s are very high and not ok for you, especially if you know that it is already on its way down. it's only bad when it stays high for hours and even worst through every other meal. I'm a type 1 diabetic and trust me 190s is not high, depending on how tired you are, your stress level, and indeed how insulin resistant you are. That will keep your sugar level high irrespective of if you have calculated how many and what type of carbs you've eaten. It's easier to manage, though you exaggerate how that cereal can kill, and not now that you know how to take care of your easier type 2 diabetes. You don't have it as bad as you proclaim to. the only reason you fainted was because of you were inexperienced, once you know how to control your consumption,

Leo M.

In four months, I have lost 62 lbs. Intermittent fasting and low carb is the key.

Sugar is the real enemy. I am down to 239.1, whereas before I did this diet, I was 302 lbs. My HGA1C now is 5.0

Kitty W

My husband was just diagnosed with insulin-dependent diabetes yesterday. The hospital didn't give him any information only needles & a meter. So your site is helping me to help him understand how serious the ailment is. Please pray for us. Thank you again.

Jane F

It is such a shame, that our Medical Community tells us NOT to eat fats!! Plus, don't eat eggs!!! And, that your cholesterol shouldn't be high. Plus don't drink whole milk! My husband is on Metaphormin, Insulin. High Blood pressure too. Cholesterol needed for our cells. Listening to them I am now tremendously Saddened for my husband and me the nagger. I am trying to save him for them. Despite doing all the doctors wanted us to do my husband has had multiple amputations. Heartbreaking!

Brotha Y.

I am now using Irish moss bladderwrack as my vitamins 3x a day as I have stopped using synthetic multivitamins prescribed by my doctor. This is the best decision I ever did. I am enjoying lots of natural energy. I can tell the big difference no more sore knees, especially when working out.

Dale Val

I'm now learning, and I feel I'm already in danger at 60, I hope God gives me more time to catch up. But if he doesn't, at least I heard some truth, and not the lies the Diabetes Association and my doctor fed me. I wish I had known this stuff 25 years ago.

Annette Fowler

I have been doing fasting and keto, and I have no more diabetes lost 30 kilos.

Uriah C

My story is very alike. Blood pressure, High sugar, cholesterol, noodles and hot dogs for dinner and eating a package of cookies a day, I usually used to feel like I wanted to pass out often and started to get confused a bit. I made up my mind to get rid of refined carbs, processed foods, and sweets. I eliminated all the junk foods including inflammatory oils, and I started an organic diet along with and proper supplements. But spoilt myself a bit over the weekends by allowing myself to eat anything I wanted. Within two months, my pants had dropped severely and did not fit anymore, and I also ran out of adjustment on all my belts. I had lost about 25 pounds in about three months even though I wasn't even trying to lose weight.

After three months of dieting, I went to my Cardiologist as I had not seen a physician in more than eight years. My Ecco stress test came back with a fantastic result, despite not taking any type of medication for those eight years. And he had said to me back then that I was in the 100 percentile range of being insulin-resistant. I'm now 65 years old. I am no longer having prediabetes with my A1c reading at 5.0. Total Cholesterol 163, and PSA from 1.0 down to 0.4. My blood pressure is not bad being in the range of 122/70, 116/76, 122/74. My triglycerides are down to 69, LDL 97, HDL 51, My mind is much sharper, and I don't even miss the foods that I used to eat. The best thing is that arthritis I had for the past 25 years is gone.

Keep in mind that I've been eating junk foods and taking no medicines of any kind for the past eight years. My doctor told me over 18 years ago that since I wasn't able to change my lifestyle, I would have to take medicines. For years I was on five different types. Today, thankfully, due to diet change, supplements, and sound advice freely and generously published, I am medicine free.

Takeaway: Don't let people convince you that you can't improve your health in a short time by eating correctly, taking some supplements, and getting minimal exercise. I'm living proof.

Shamil C

So true, diet, diet and no medications. When you got used to your new diet, you will never crave the high carb. I completely reversed my Type 2 diabetes, and my doctor has stopped prescribing metformin & glyburide for me.

Ortiz M

I had fasting of 180 took my kid to work came back had a cup of black coffee and tested again after two hours and my fasting sugar was still at 179. I am hungry so had three eggs with a spoon of butter well not real butter and a handful of raw spinach cooked. Then will retest again in an hour or two. I feel more stable when sugar is 180 vs. 200s. My motivation level is increased, and my head is clearer. I am still not on metformin as am yet to pick up from the pharmacy but holy moly my sugar is just not coming down not been under 130 in weeks, am wondering if water fast could help.

Rose M

For a week now, I have been on the low carb diet. My blood sugar has been fluctuating between 101 to 109, I ate a little bit of Cheerios this morning, and one-third cup of heavy whipping cream plus one cup of water with my fasting sugar level at 108. One hour After eating the Cheerios, my fasting blood sugar was a whopping 208. No more cereal for me! My system can't handle grains of any kinds, nor any sort of milk.

Jeanne W.

When my blood sugar gets high after a high carb meal, it takes Hours and hours to drop back down.

KADI D

God bless you all; reversing diabetes is a reality. I have done it.

Honey H

I am not diagnosed with diabetes yet, but all the women in my family have it. My mum died from Lipitor side effects when she had Alzheimer's. So I need to prevent this future deadly disease. Thank you.

James L

Thank you. I don't want to be on medication; so I have changed the way I eat. As described. I went from high 300ths to a so-called normal average of 120. A1C of 13.9 to 5.0 in about four months. Eat to live. God bless you all.

Brian N

Walking after meals might also help, especially with LCHF, Elimination Diet, and intermittent fasting. Perhaps the proverb is correct: 100 steps after meals, and live 99 years.

Arazim S

Eating outside does no good. Veges is the answer. Never get more than 70% full.

Ricky Maynard

I have been labeled a person with diabetes in the last couple of years, but not on medication. My A1C kept creeping up to 7.0, and my doctor threatened to put me on metformin. I told her to give me two months, but she graciously gave me four months. I cut out all bread, and all potatoes, and anything with high carbs at all I have dropped 16lbs. In 40 days, and I am still staying the course, with hopes of breaking 199lbs in a few weeks. Today I weigh 203 down from 219. I have two months to go before I am tested again. I think

I can safely say my A1C will be 6.0 or below. Thanks to you for helping me see the light.

Andrea L

I have seen that book. I'm an "O" too. I'm following this because my blood sugar was 471. It scared me needless to say.

Malone K

Doctors test blood sugar levels but don't check insulin levels. People show acceptable blood sugar levels (sub 100) for years but have all the other indicators of metabolic syndrome indicating high circulating insulin that continually has to drive the blood sugar under 100. Suddenly the sugar count rises and can't be kept under 100 and voila! You have type 2 diabetes. That's why fasting and low carb are so essential to driving insulin down as many hours per day as possible. This assuages the fatty liver and causes organ fat to be used up for energy needs, and weight loss follows along with blood pressure and other metabolic indicators.

Sharon M

They told me, "once you damage any part of your insides from diabetes it's permanent." Once you reverse Type 2 and bounce back to a healthy lifestyle how do you restore other issues, if any, that was caused by having Type 2?

Carolyn M

Lots of people do want to change their habits. The problem is they are already addicted. People can appreciate that they can get addicted to drugs, alcohol cigarettes, and even sex, but they have little no understanding about being addicted to sugar and carbs. That is why so many regularly "fall off the wagon" because there's an addiction in the body. Food is everywhere. We must eat, but we don't have to smoke or drink alcohol. So I understand this addiction more because it's everywhere. Carbs and sugars are everywhere! I'm sick of it. The glucose meter is the real deal!!

Gonzalez A.

The metformin was my excuse to eat a little of this or a bit of that when I couldn't stop eating carbs. I am done feeling guilty about what I eat. So I started Keto 90 days ago, and I have lost 20 lbs. I am going for blood work next week. I am excited as I look forward to seeing the outcome.

Manuel I.

First and foremost I want to praise the "most high" my Lord Jesus Christ. Special thanks to Ken for sharing his story. My name is Manuel. I'm thirty-nine years old. Four years ago, I was diagnosed with type 2 diabetes. In my 20s through my mid-30s all my Physicians always said I was pre-diabetic and that I needed to work on trying to bring my weight down but end up going back to my old habits. I have been on a seesaw weight loss from 289 to 251. Two hundred and eighty-nine being the highest I've ever weighed and two hundred and fifty-one being the lowest I have weighed in the last ten years. For someone that weighed 147 in high school because I played football, I was in Reserve Officer Training Corps and did Physical Education. I now weigh 261. I never thought I would be diabetic which I believe is a lousy mixture of over drinking alcohol, eating fast foods and no exercising routinely landed me where I am now. Three years ago I got married to most beautiful God loving woman I have ever known, and we now have two little boys Donny who's turning 2 and Ezra who's four months old. Our Lord Jesus says that everything is possible through him and I believe this to be true. In the last month, my sugar level has been as high as 485 and as low as 197. Before following you, I was already determined to turn my life around to make life-changing Lifestyles for the Love of my wife and my two baby boys so that I could see them grow up into God-loving men. I believe that following you, was a positive sign from God to me. Thank you for sharing your experience.

AmeriJam A

My fiancé had an A1C of 11.4, and after seven weeks the app I use to track her glucose estimates an A1C of 7.5.

Junlyn L

My blood sugar goes up to 462, but I lower to 156 after two weeks. Just manage your food intake. I always recommend one bulb of sliced garlic every morning. I wish I could be more helpful for people like us.

Sky Runner

I had the same experience you had, and you have explained every aspect fantastically well. The biggest problem I had was my doctor freaking when my Total Cholesterol and low-density lipoproteins LDL went up initially although my Triglycerides/HDL ratio, HbA1c, Fasting Insulin, and Inflammation marker plummeted to better than "normal." Getting the Cholesterol culprit exposed and Medical Profession reformed is now one of the essential pre-requisites to allow Type-2 Diabetics to reverse on the Low-Carb Healthy Fat Lifestyle or Keto with the full support of Medical Profession and Insurers who still use the meaningless Total Cholesterol as a criterion.

Robert N

I went from A1C of 13 to 6.8. And I'm still working on it. Changing from sugar to fat for energy is like going from diesel to jet fuel.

Tony G

For me, it's easy as water. Chicken breast broccoli. It gets old, but it works.

Stewart T

Eighteen months ago, when I was 31 years old, I had no diabetic symptoms other than slow healing from injuries. I went to the hospital believing I had Lyme disease from a tick bite (which by the way, I also tested positive for) that had gotten infected, but they told me I had diabetes too. It happened to be a morning appointment, so I was fasting, and my Fasting blood sugar was 351. I didn't look overweight, because I was muscular due to the nature of my job being physical. I started keto diet about 4 or 5 months ago, and I have lost about 30 lbs (mostly water weight from what I can tell - inflammation) and my Fasting blood sugar when I check it now is always between 90-100. I was placed on, metformin and then Januvia medication but the metformin didn't change my Fasting blood sugar, and as such didn't seem to help that much. I have a new appointment with my physician coming up soon, so I'm curious to see what my A1C will be. At my first appointment a year and a half ago it was over 11. It is sad knowing that my entire life I was avoiding fats, and eating a ton of carbs because I was always told that was the way to live. It's crazy to think I was not only poisoning myself the entire time with carbs but simultaneously denying my body the fat it needed.

Tman Y

I lost my twin brother In 2009 to a heart attack due to Harding of the artery's, and he had diabetes. Soon after I had a quad bypass and just recently got diagnosed with type 2 diabetes. In 2 months I brought my A1C down from 8.0 to 5.8 and my weight from 280lbs to 240lbs by cutting carbs with green juice fasting, and intermittent fasting.

Ain A

God did say that knowledge will increase in the last days and there it is folks. Keto and other low carbs diet are a big blessing from God and don't be afraid to get some help from God and all good people on the information pipeline. Many good brothers and sisters are out there, study, research, and learn that you are what you eat

K Haenga

I got diagnosed over two years now, and I feel like I am losing control. I have always subscribed to the notion of a little bit is ok. But I know this has created the worst problem for me. Changing my diet has been so difficult, but now I am convinced I must do it or face the result of taking things for granted.

Thank you. This is the motivation I needed to change. I just turned 50 and am experiencing all the symptoms - poor eyesight, dry throat, frequent urination, and I hope it's not too late.

David H

My A1C was 14.5 but three months into a Keto diet it has gone down to 6. Also lost 12kg (26pound) within the period, feel great.

John V

My A1C was 9.0 the day I was diagnosed but presently am in 5.4 after seven months of being diagnosed

Natalee S

I have been off medications for two years now because I changed my eating habits. It is now, no processed foods, no sugar, and low carbs.

Tracy B

I love cereal, and It is impossible for me not to eat any sweets. I do eat healthier and will practice intermittent fasting. I shall continue to take Gymnema, and ashwagandha and I am going to drink fenugreek water.

Dahlia S

People with diabetes that have developed kidney issues have to follow a low purine diet also. Most of the low glycemic veggies would set off gout attacks. Thank God for allopurinol.

Warren D

I think fruit and whole grain is one of the worst offenders for people living with diabetes. Most doctors all around push eating whole grain garbage and fruits. Both are awful!

Dolly A

Thank you for this. I just heard someone I love with all my heart has diabetes type 2 with more than 500 blood glucose. Trying to learn all we can to lower it.

Megan T

To alleviate my having Type 2 diabetes and addiction to carbs like spaghetti, I acquired a veggie spiralizer. I investigated different brands and bought "The Veggetti Pro" and is so simple to work. I now use 2-3 packs of spaghetti to make low carb noodles from spaghetti." (You have to heat them to soften them). Then you put sauce and other things as well. Amazing, I got the table top one: in the yellow box (simple to use & clean and has the suction to the table) Don't get the lower priced handheld ones (hard to work). Anyway, this product converts recipes with high carbs into healthy low carbs. It's like you are cheating, but it tastes great! Plus you can use lots of other low carb veggies to do all sorts of things as well. Don't use a potato though. Just too many carbs.

Trucka M

My A1C went up to 7 from 6.2. I have to get it down. I'm on 1000mg metformin, but it gives me gas frequently, but they do have a time discharge version (1000 mg metformin E.R.). Keep away from glucosamine although it helps lower your A1C because mine used to be 8.4 but the glucosamine causes weight gain, and I'm fat enough, so I stop taking it. I need suggestions for any remedies, thank you.

Blooze D

Mine was 11.3 when I was diagnosed. Some charts online didn't even go that high. I think that translated to about 345 on a test strip. I got it down to 6.7 after three months then down within the low 5s after six months. It's quite simple don't eat high carb foods even "healthy" ones according to the geniuses at the America Diabetes Association.

John H

I need to do this. I am addicted to sugar. I was a smoker; I did quit that. I can do this! I will quit sugar! Right now. I will miss the sugar, But I like veggies and fats so maybe this will help me leave the sugar! I will stop the sugar.

Lirek R

Thanks for sharing the information. I have type 2 diabetes, and any time I try to fast (like one meal a day) I do have low blood sugar,

Grandpa F

Unfortunately, governments are not doing much to enlighten people and promote eating less sugar and carbs because of the implications of trillions of dollars in the drug and food industries. It will also affect governments who have put in trillions of dollars in the medical sectors. Thinking of how much these governments will suffer a loss if people are curing themselves using this method. There is a smearing campaign going on to put off people from curing themselves of diabetes and probably cancer.

Bob L

I was diagnosed at 16.1 and instructed: "do not go to the internet looking for miracle cures; all we can do is to control the disease."

So I went to the internet, and they will give you a far better explanation of essential facts you need to find out from a physician and will also not hand you over to the pharmaceutical industry. Intermittent fasting with a Ketogenic diet reduces your blood glucose, but it requires about three to four weeks of changing over from carb burning to fat burning. I have better energy; and if you do not feel hungry, then Intermittent Fasting is easy to do. However, my low-density lipoprotein (LDL) cholesterol is up. Far higher than what is considered allowable, and another item for me to work on.

Christine S

So, you can eat cereal if you're careful. For me, the secret is to put it in plain almond based yogurt. It's one carb per 1/3 cup. I use math and my scale to measure out ten carbs portion of a high fiber cereal like fiber one or sola brand granola. I add five carbs portion of fruit. My blood sugar doesn't budge.

Also, your lentil soup recipe gave me the courage to try adding beans back. I now can enjoy black bean soup, lentil soup, and chili.

If you have any information on appropriate preparation for disasters, I'd be interested in the assistance. The recent NC hurricane made me find out how carbohydrate high food choices are if you can't cook stuff up. I lived on nuts, seeds, a limited quantity of fruit and veggies, and stable shelf diabetes-friendly meal alternative shakes for three days. I can't say I wasn't tempted to grab stuff like chips, but I left them for the girls.

McNabb R

I have 13-14 A1C for more than one year. I am now trying a ketogenic diet and without family support.

Roger L

I went to the physician yesterday my A1C was 6.4 that raise by one point, and I added weight so am back to testing. I have been drinking fruit and veggie blends. I tested this morning about half an hour after I ate my breakfast and it was 131. An hour after that was 168 no more juice for me now they want me to take glucose tolerance test the reason is because of agent orange so back to watching my carbs.

Tweeny D

I have reasonable control of my diabetes with the help of metformin plus the diet and exercise.

Cristian S

As of October 23, 2018, my A1C was 6.5, so I was legally a person living with diabetes. As of today, I am 25lbs less, and my A1C is 5.7. In 3 months I have cut all high carbs such as pasta, rice, potato, bread, sweet fruits, and sugars. My triglycerides were 313 in the past and 101 today. I feel happy doing intermittent fasting.

Liberty M

I have searched the internet and cannot get a straight-forward answer from anyone on how to transition off of insulin once you have gone keto or carnivore and have commenced intermittent fasting. This is the dilemma I am having: Insulin in the fat storage hormone. Yes, it lowers your blood glucose, but it does it by just pulling the glucose out of your blood and storing it somewhere else in your body as fat. So how can I reduce my weight if I keep injecting insulin into my body? I suspended my injections for a few days, and my blood glucose raised again, but I reduced my weight. It's like a catch 22. Stay fat, take your insulin and have good device numbers or you stop taking insulin, let your levels increase, and reduce your weight. What do I do? This is driving me crazy! Please, someone, explain this to me. Thanks.

David S.

I experience the "Dawn effect" frequently, I can eat a small piece of meat or an egg, and it brings it down to an average level, so for me, it's all about test, test, test, and tests some more, your meter is your best friend.

Zacarias L.

I am in the middle to upper 4's (86 in USA scale) of the blood sugar scale; if I take slow acting carbs (not keto diet per se), when I overeat. I get to 5.2 or 5,3 (93-94 in USA scale). I do trek about 4 kilometers with a vested weight of 40 pounds and have maximum energy; and yes, I cannot eat fruits either, LoL. God bless you all.

Maria J.

Some months ago whenever I had a reading of 150 or higher, I would cry. Now if that happens, I just alter what I eat. I have discovered it is an ever-changing situation. I am excited to say in the past month my highest result was 155, but that was a dawn effect so one high reading in 30 days, I am delighted with that result.

Charles M.

My blood sugar was 8.0 without medication and 7.0 with medication. I stopped all medicines when I started the low carbohydrate, high-fat diet. For three months now, I have been eating low carb high-fat diet.

My three-month checkup shows my A1C has come down from 8.0 to 6.0

David G.

There is nothing wrong with a 4.9. I suspended one of my medications when I began intermittent fasting, and I dropped to 4.8, and my doctor was happy and cut my other medication in half, hoping to end it for good within the next thirty days.

Kenneth Y.

The dawn effect was one of the tools my doctor used to verify the diagnosis of diabetes, along with the A1C, which was his first tool. I reversed my diabetes with a ketogenic diet and intermittent fasting. My doctor's prescription was a low glucose, low fat, instead of my suggested course of very low-carb and, the disciplined form of intermittent fasting. He was unfamiliar with my suggestion. These are the diabetic's best tools to manage insulin and blood glucose naturally, by clearing the fatty liver that presents the biggest challenge, along with dysfunctional mitochondria in the cells.

Martlamb M.

The Dawn Effect is a Phenomenon caused by your liver making glucose in the early morning hours in preparation for your body to wake up. Eating anything makes your pancreas release insulin then your sugar levels return to lower levels. I started keto/carnivore in Jan with fasting sugar numbers around 230. Medications just made me gain weight, so I stopped taking them. Today my fasting sugar is 156, and I have dropped 33 pounds. It is all God's doing. He takes away my cravings, my hunger, and my food addictions. To God be all the glory. I thank Him daily.

Lee J.

Doctors just don't want you to eat anything lol. But I received great news today from my doctor. I reduced my A1C level significantly and dropped over 15 pounds. I eat healthier and fast intermittently, but I didn't cut off everything. I either eat smaller amounts (like carbs) or find other ways to consume better foods.

Robert H

I am a single dad who just discovered at the beginning of December that I had diabetes. My blood glucose was 377 and A1C was 10.9. I started medication while charting everything I ate and walking a few days a week. But I did as you say test, test, test. Last week my A1C was 5.1, and I tried hard to keep blood sugar between 90 to 120. But no pasta, rice, or bread. 90% of what I eat is fresh vegetables. I have lost up to 40 lbs.

Catalina C.

My grandma lived up to 93 and ate a lot of homemade sausages. She raised chickens and had her vegetable garden. She also ate some bread; she baked herself and some wine. She ate lunch and a tiny dinner with one boiled egg). She avoided many fruits.

Michael H

I just got diagnosed today with type 2 diabetics. A1c at 11.3. I thought I was having eye issues because things got blurry, turns out as if it was just the sugar level that was high.about.270 before today I didn't even know what sugar was or did, just that it sweetened my cereal. Until last week I craved Coke like water and one or two liters every two days was regular, for years. Now it's time to get back on course. Please pray for me. Eyes at 20/25 and blood pressure steady at 125/83.

Ricky B.

It never stops to perplex me how the so-called medical professionals keep insisting on a low-fat, high in carbohydrates diet when there is now so much proof that the reverse is true.

Dragan S

I moved from an A1C 14 and dropped it down to 5.1 in three months. I was taking cholesterol, insulin, and blood pressure medications. I went from a glucose level of 250 to 80. I dropped all the pills and lost 70 pounds. I exercise five days a week, and I could appear in a fitness magazine. I was off work for two months due to the diabetes complication. Here I am 1 year after healthier than ever. All things are indeed possible if you put your mind to it.

Natural Treatment using Herbs

The conventional treatment approach for diabetes entails the dosing of insulin.

Diabetes is a disease characterized by the excessive presence of sugar in human blood. So whatever treatment approach should be aimed at controlling the blood sugar or reducing it whenever it rises beyond usual. So it is for this reason that standard medical practice utilizes the injection of insulin to try reducing the blood sugar. For type 1 diabetes, this drug administration is in order except for a drastic drop resulting in low blood sugar. However, the application of insulin in type2 diabetes is paradoxically wrong considering that this form of diabetic is already suffering from an excessive amount of insulin in their bloodstream. This is the reason why the treatment approach with drugs has been very ineffective over so many decades of this practice.

An alternative treatment approach using herbal medicine offers a safe and more effective treatment with a high possibility of reversing diabetes. The use of herbs entails the application of natural foods, seeds, and leaves. Cases of overdose are rare because the body handles them like any other food or fruit we consume. Nobody measures the number of apples consumed daily, but we all know when to reduce intake such as when we experience any adverse body reaction like stooling.

I like the way Dr. Fung explains the cause of both types of diabetes. He says "type 1 diabetes is due to inadequate insulin in the body, while type 2 diabetes is the result of excess insulin. But paradoxically doctors continue to prescribe an increased dosage of insulin as treatment." And I ask, why do doctors treat a disease with more and more dosage of its causative agent. We all know that dietary shortcomings cause both type 1 and type 2 diabetes. So isn't wise and instructive that our treatment program for both types of diabetes should be focused on diet improvement or changes.

There are now more far-reaching methods of reversing type 2 diabetes.

The Newcastle Diet research, which entailed eating six hundred calories per day for eight weeks, led to seven of eleven participants being free from type 2 diabetes. MRI scans showed the diet led to fat reduction within the liver and pancreas of participants which resulted in notably improved blood sugar levels.

After three months, the seven participants, that had become free from type 2 diabetes, had returned to regularly eating after receiving advice on eating portion size and healthily. All of them have been able to stay off medication.

One of the limits of the Newcastle Diet, however, was its small size. This is the reason Diabetes UK are currently funding their biggest ever research project into an ultra-low calorie liquid diet, and its ability to send type 2 diabetes into long-term remission.

Another remarkable method of reversing type 2 diabetes is bariatric surgery, which can be done through procedures such as gastric banding or. gastric bypass

An American study recently discovered that obese type 2 diabetes patients had higher reversal following weight-loss surgery than those who implemented lifestyle changes alone. However, a 2011 research investigating bariatric surgery found that 62 percent of gastric banding patients and 83 percent of gastric bypass patients were off their type 2 medication after two years. However, only 36 percent maintained normal blood sugar levels without diabetes medication after ten years. This study seems to contradict the earlier study that inferred that surgery was more beneficial than lifestyle changes alone.

Most weight-loss procedures involve patients maintaining a strict diet before and after the surgery, to ensure long-term reversal.

While the weight loss can reverse type 2 diabetes, however, it is sustaining disciplined dietary improvements that will keep the condition reversed for several years after the surgery.

That is what matters with regards to reversing type 2 diabetes in the long-term.

Whether you commit to lifestyle interventions, have weight-loss surgery, or use the Newcastle diet, a tremendous amount of hard work and commitment is needed to avoid falling back into bad habits.

5.1 Herbal Remedies

Herbal Tea

Researchers have attributed the health properties of tea to polyphenols (a type of antioxidant) and phytochemicals. Ginger tea is a spicy and flavor-rich drink that packs a punch of healthy, disease-fighting antioxidants. While green tea is more often linked with antioxidants, white tea contains more antioxidants. Peppermint tea is one of the most commonly used herbal teas in the world. The peppermint oil is a well known essential oil. Peppermint oil is a versatile essential oil and may be applied topically, internally and aromatically to address a lot of health concerns, such as muscles aches and seasonal allergy symptoms, low energy and digestive complaints. It's also commonly used to improve both skin and hair health and boost energy levels.

Additionally, studies have shown that drinking tea is appropriate for your health; teas can help protect your heart, and your teeth as well as possibly lower the risk of cancer, can help lower blood pressure and it can encourage weight loss.

Tumeric

This is a piece of the ginger family, it has a strong smell, and distinctive orange color (which distinguishes it from Ginger) and for which the chemical curcumin is responsible, are instantly recognizable. Turmeric is a favorite seasoning in Traditional African and Indian recipes. You can find this herbal medicine in all supermarkets for cooking and health food stores as supplements.

This is one herb, more effective than anything else to heal inflammation diseases such as type 2 diabetes. And not only does it decreases inflammation, but it has also been proven to treat the pancreas cells damaged by type 2 diabetes, aside from its anti-inflammatory properties, which have been broadly studied. Turmeric contains a chemical called aromatic turmerone, which has been discovered to repair stem cells. You can also take turmerone as a supplement seen in all health food stores.

Curcumin present in Turmeric might help to handle diabetes by improving blood sugar as good as insulin levels. Turmeric would also reverse cell damage such as wounds, kidney damage, and ulcers that are associated with diabetes. This is due to its antioxidant and anti-inflammatory properties.

This offers a punch or two to the damage inflammation causes to beta cells in the pancreas, which have responsibility for the production of insulin. Not only do the anti-inflammatory agents ward off damaging free radicals, but any damage already done is repaired by the aromatic turmerone.

HOW TO MAKE TUMERIC DRINKS

a) Turmeric Amla Juice

Take a quarter (1/4) teaspoon of Turmeric powder. Put and shake it in 10 cl of Amla juice. Indian gooseberry or amla is without a doubt a powerhouse of nutrients. One of the beneficial ways to add amla to your diet is to make juice out of it. As with any useful health food, there can also be some adverse side effects. If you consume too much Tumeric-amla juice, you might experience allergic reactions, dry skin, hypoglycemia, acid reflux, hypotension, and constipation.

So, drink it once daily 2 hours after your meal. Do this for one or two (1-2) months for best results.

b) Tumeric Tea

Add half a teaspoonful of turmeric powder to one teaspoonful of any of the herbal tea suggested above (Peppermint tea, Ginger tea, Green tea, and White tea) and take it twice a day for 30/45 days.

Milk Thistle

Milk thistle is a biennial or annual plant of the Asteraceae family. Milk thistle has other common names including Silybum marianum, Carduus marianus, Marian thistle, Mary thistle, blessed milk thistle, Holy thistle, Saint Mary's thistle, Scotch thistle, variegated thistle, and Mediterranean milk thistle. Silymarin, an active ingredient in milk thistle, acts as an antioxidant by reducing free radical production.

Milk thistle is often taken as a natural treatment for liver problems. These liver issues include gallbladder disorders, jaundice, hepatitis, and cirrhosis. Milk thistle also Provide heart benefits by lowering cholesterol levels and help reduce the effect of diabetes in people who have cirrhosis and type 2 diabetes. Studies have shown a reduction in blood glucose levels and an improvement in cholesterol in people with type 2 diabetes. Medical research does suggest that milk thistle, together with traditional treatment, can improve diabetes. Researchers have also inferred that milk thistle improved insulin resistance, a key characteristic of type 2 diabetes.

Side effects of milk thistle include; Diarrhea, Allergic reactions, Abdominal bloating/pain, Gas, Indigestion, Itching, Loss of appetite and Nausea.

Milk thistle is available as a powder, liquid extract, and capsule. The recommended dosage is a total of 420 mg per day. Every capsule should contain at least 70 percent silymarin. Please note that taking milk thistle with diabetes drugs might cause additive effects.

HOW TO MAKE MILK THISTLE DRINKS

Step1: Dry some milk thistle seeds and ground to powder.

Step 2: Get an empty tea bag and fill a tea with the powdered milk thistle.

Step 3: Place the tea bag in a cup and pour some hot in it

Step 4: Leave the tea bag in hot water for 3-5 minutes.

Step 5: Strain the tea bag, and enjoy!

Dandelion

Dandelion is an herb also known as Wild Endive, Taraxaci Herba, Taraxacum, Tête de Moine, Pisse au Lit, Pissenlit, Priest's Crown, Pu Gong Ying, Salade de Taupe, Swine Snout, Florion d'Or, Fausse Chicorée, Florin d'Or, Délice Printanier, Dent-de-Lion, Diente de

Leon, Dudal, Endive Sauvage,Herba Taraxaci, Laitue de Chien, Leontodon taraxacum, Lion's Tooth, Cankerwort, Cochet, Couronne de Moine, Blowball, and other names.

The dandelion plant root may be used as a mild laxative and has been used to improve digestion. Preliminary animal studies indicate that dandelion may help normalize blood sugar levels and lower total cholesterol and triglycerides while raising HDL (good) cholesterol in mice with diabetes.

Dandelion leaves and roots have been used widely, for many years for its health and medicinal benefits. However, a systematic review of data shows a dearth of knowledge on its use as an anti-diabetic herb. Thus the purpose of the study was to determine the anti-diabetic effect of dandelion root and leaf powder in type 2 patients with diabetes. An estimated sample size of sixty (60) Type 2 diabetic patients was recruited from the diabetes center of the Komfo Anokye Teaching Hospital (KATH) in Kumasi, Ghana for the clinical study and randomly distributed into three groups. In total the first group of participants received 45 g of dandelion leaf powder, the second group received 45 g of dandelion root powder and the third group (the experiment control group) received no treatment. The first two groups (intervention groups) consumed 5 g of dandelion each day for nine days. Participants took 5 g of the remedy each day and fasting blood glucose (FBS) were tested before and during the treatment periods and recorded into data capturing sheets. The results showed that about 61% of these participants were females, 53.33% and 10% were overweight and obese respectively, and 86.7% of the study participants were between the ages of 40 and 70 years, Average caloric intakes of participants in all three groups increased over the study period but were not significant ($p > 0.05$). Consumption of 5 g of dandelion root and leaf powder for nine (9) days significantly reduced the fasting blood sugar levels from 10.7 mmol/L to 7.5 mmol/L ($p < 0.05$) and 10.5 mmol/L to 8.6 mmol/L ($p < 0.05$) respectively of type two patients with diabetes. For the control, the average FBS rose from 10.8 mmol/L to 10.9 mmol/L. However, fasting blood sugar result was not statistically significant ($p > 0.05$). There was no difference in fasting blood sugar between those who consumed the leaves and those who consumed the roots. The rate of urination was not affected significantly by the consumption of dandelion roots or leaves.

Inculcating traditional medicinal plants like dandelion into the treatment and management of diabetes may help improve the well-being and health of type 2 patients with diabetes.

Dandelion supplements are available in some health food stores and on the internet. People can also buy dandelion root tea.

Dandelion root is usually considered safe and is well tolerated in adults if consumed in moderation. Some persons might experience side effects, including diarrhea, heartburn, irritated skin and upset stomach.

Dandelion greens refer to the leaves of the dandelion and can be sautéed, steamed or even eaten raw. They possess an earthy, bitter taste and can be used in a variety of meals. On the other hand, dandelion root, is often ground into a powder and then roasted and added raw to herbal teas or used as a coffee substitute. Everything, from the dandelion flower down to the roots, is edible. And, dandelions also happen to be delicious. However, dandelion leaves, which can be eaten as a vegetable, are rich in oxalates so should be taken in moderation. The taste of dandelion is similar to bitter green like arugula. You can cook them on the stove, or eat them fresh in salads.

HOW TO MAKE DANDELION ROOT TEA

Wash the dandelion roots in fresh water. Use a soft brush to scrub the dirt off the roots. They will look entirely white and knobby. Dry the dandelion roots with some heat, natural sunlight or in an oven, until crisp and hard. Store in a glass jar, The properly dried roots will stay preserved for a year or more when kept in a dry and cool place.

Dandelion root tea is a decoction, not an infusion. Crush the dandelion root in a mortar until it is chunky, and the size of lentils (about 5mm). Place the root in a pan, put some water and simmer on the stove for about 15 minutes. Allow the decoction to settle, and then strain it into your cup.

Licorice root

The root of Glycyrrhiza glabra which has a pleasant taste is what we refer to as Licorice root. The licorice plant is native to southern

Europe, parts of Asia and the Middle East such as India; and is a perennial herbaceous legume

Researchers at the Max Planck Institution for Molecular Genetics in Berlin have now found out that licorice root also contains substances with an anti-diabetic effect. These amorfruitins are very well tolerated; they not only decrease blood glucose, but they are also anti-inflammatory and. It is mostly administered in the form of tea and has been used in traditional healing for millennia. Licorice root is the raw material for licorice candy

WARNING: Drinking Licorice tea for longer than 7 days can cause potentially dangerous adverse side effects. Please do not drink licorice tea for over a week without taking a break for some weeks.

Ensure you only get licorice root that does not have glycyrrhizin; which is referred to as DGL or deglycyrrhizinated licorice. Large doses of Glycyrrhizin can interfere with normal adrenal function, as well as cause water retention and leg swell up.

Because of how powerful this herb is, I usually advise that you don't use licorice tea without your doctor's approval.

HOW TO PREPARE LICORICE ROOT TEA

Boil four to eight ounces of water in a pot, depending on how much tea you want to make.

Place one teaspoon of dried licorice root into the pot for every 4 ounces of water.

Let out the water from the heat and let the licorice root steep in the pot for 5 minutes.

Pour the tea through a fine-mesh kitchen sieve set over a teacup or a teapot. Then you can discard the dried licorice root.

Fenugreek

Fenugreek is a herb that can also be used to control diabetes, improve sugar tolerance and lower blood glucose levels as a result of its hypoglycaemic activity.

Soak two tablespoons of fenugreek seeds in water over the night. Consume the water together with the seeds when the day breaks on an empty stomach. Follow this preparation without fail for a few months to bring down your sugar level.

On the alternative, it is recommended that you take two tablespoons of powdered fenugreek seeds every day with milk.

Fenugreek seeds can assist reduce the risk of developing diabetes. Fenugreek seeds have galactomannan and essential amino acids.

Galactomannan brings down blood glucose level, and essential amino acids improve insulin level in the blood. Together, this helps in controlling diabetes.

HOW TO MAKE FENUGREEK DRINKS TEA

a) Fenugreek Tea

Take 1 or 2 teaspoons of Fenugreek seeds.

Boil the seeds in a cup of water for 10 minutes, then

sieve to remove the water from the seeds. And allow the water to cool through the night.

Drink the Fenugreek water on an empty stomach in the morning. Take this Fenugreek tea 1-2 times a day.

Continue this for 1-2 months for better results.

b) Fenugreek Seeds Capsule

Take 1-2 Fenugreek capsules.

Consume it with water after taking your meals two times a day

Cinnamon

According to a current review study by researchers from Western University of Health Sciences in Pomona, California, a very well-known herb, often used in desserts, cakes and pies have a fantastic ability to tackle type 2 diabetes.

Also, this spice promotes cardiovascular health by reducing harmful LDL cholesterol and triglycerides in the blood.

In the recent review study, investigators analyzed results of 10 randomized control lead studies of cinnamon's effects on diabetes patients. Studies involved five hundred and forty-three participants, all having type 2 diabetes and compared two groups; one that took no herbal remedy, and the other that took a cinnamon remedy for a period of four to eighteen weeks. The daily dose of a cinnamon remedy ranged from 120 milligrams to 6 grams.

After collating the results, study investigators discovered a significant improvement in blood glucose and cholesterol levels in study participants who took the supplement. Their fasting sugar levels were reduced by an impressive 25 milligrams/deciliter.

Researchers state that the secret benefits of cinnamon lie in a powerful compound called cinnamaldehyde, which can control and stimulate the effects of insulin.

Improved insulin sensitivity lowers blood glucose levels, drastically improving type 2 diabetes.

According to studies, the same substance is responsible for the cardiovascular potentials of cinnamon. It has been noted that cinnamon supplements did curtail not only "bad" LDL cholesterol but also increased the levels of HDL, or "good" cholesterol.

However, make sure that you get the best quality cinnamon powder or supplements since many types of "cinnamon" sold in supermarkets and online shops are more like sawdust and include almost no cinnamon.

But taking cinnamon is only one piece of the puzzle when it comes to healing type 2 diabetes. Powdered cinnamon can reduce blood glucose levels by triggering insulin activity. It contains bioactive components that can help prevent and fight diabetes.

Take three to five capsules of Cinnamon powder daily. Do not take the same time as regular medications, and allow two hours apart.

HOW TO MAKE CINNAMON DRINKS TEA

You can add cinnamon to warm beverages, smoothies, and baked goods. Put around one teaspoon of cinnamon powder in a cup of warm water, mix and drink daily. Alternatively, boil two to four cinnamon sticks in a cup of water and allow it to steep for twenty minutes, then drink this daily until you see improvement.

Bitter Gourd

Bitter gourd commonly called bitter melon can be helpful for controlling diabetes due to its blood glucose lowering effects. It tends to influence glucose metabolism across your body instead of just a particular tissue or organ. It is recommended that you drink some bitter gourd juice on an empty stomach each morning.

HOW TO MAKE BITTER GOURD DRINKS TEA

First, remove the seeds from one or more bitter gourds, then extract the juice using a juicer. You can add some water and then drink it.

Do this daily in the morning for at least two months as a treatment.

You can also include one dish made of bitter gourd daily in your diet.

5.2 How To Make 4-in 1 Herbal Capsule

I will be giving you details of how to make potent herbal medicine at home in capsule form. This is to ensure that you don't end up buying plain chalk instead of the actual intended herbal remedy.

Before taking this medicine, it is strongly advised that you should have corrected your diet choice to a whole food set. Depending on your body mass index, swallow two or three capsules of this 4 in 1 herb daily after meal. Allow two (2) hours apart, as it is not recommended that you take this herbal capsule at the same time of taking other doctor prescribed drugs.

First, let's look at how to prepare medicines by placing powder forms of our herbal products into capsules for easy consumption.

You will require empty capsules to fill your powders at desired potencies, thereby avoiding tablet binders and fillers. For instance "00" gelatin capsules should hold around 700-900 mg of most vitamin powders.

WHAT YOU WILL NEED

i)   Capping Machine: A capping machine and empty gelatin capsules. "The Cap-M-Quick" can cap 50 capsules at a time, but you have to manually join the capsule ends together whereas "The Capsule Machine" can only do 24 capsules at a time. Both machines can use either size 0 or size 00 capsules. However, 'the capsule machine' joins the capsule ends together automatically.

ii)   Milligram Scale: You need a milligram scale to weigh your powders. Note that a milligram scale with 1mg accuracy is essential for this manufacturing exercise.

iii)   Herbal powders for your blend. A filler material used to fill the unused space in your capsules that your active compound did not fill. Some suggested powders include corn starch, baking soda, glutamine, flour creatine, etc.

iv)   A pestle and mortar to thoroughly mix your herbs and filler.

v)   Empty Gel Capsules

5.3 How To Make Your Capsule Blends

For this demonstration, we will assume you are using The Capsule Machine. So load 24 empty capsules into your capsule machine and fill them with your preferred filler.

Weigh the filler powder after removing the filler from the capsule machine then to get the weight of the filler ingredient per capsule, divide the weight obtained earlier by the number of capsules.

Next, obtain the weight of your active compound per capsule by repeating the above steps.

LET'S ESTIMATE YOUR SUPPLEMENTS' RATIO:

In some cases, you will need to determine the ratio between your supplements to dose your compounds accurately. We will be mixing glutamine (the filler) with equal quantities of four herbs (turmeric, milk thistle, Licorice, and dandelion) which are the active compounds. Baking soda is excellent also as a filler for diabetes remedies, as such could be used in place of glutamine.

Use the measuring cup that comes with most syrup drugs to measure equal quantities of each of turmeric, milk thistle, Licorice, and dandelion root powder; then thoroughly mix all together.

Now determine how many grams of the powder of the mixed herb that is contained in one capsule. This can easily be ascertained by filling a capsule with the mixed herbs and weighing it then subtract the weight of an empty capsule.

So, to obtain the weight of mixed herbs powder required to fill 48 capsules you multiply the weight of one capsule by 24.

MIX YOUR FILLER AND YOUR ACTIVE COMPOUND

If you have pre-specified weights of the various herbs and they don't add up to the total weight that the capsule size can hold, then it becomes evident that you will need to add a filler to make up the shortfall.

But for our four in one mixed herbs, using a "oo" gelatine capsule, there wouldn't be the need for a filler. The "oo" gelatin capsule holds an average of 700-900 of powder turmeric. And we will be consuming about 200mg daily of each of the four herbs bringing the total weight of the four herbs desired to about 800mg. So we know that a mixed portion of the four herbs when filled in the capsule, will amount to our desired target of about 800mg.

Now you are set to produce your first capsules!

CAPSULE FILLER MACHINE INSTRUCTIONS:

If you have never made nootropic capsules before, following the instructions above may be intimidating.

1. To mix and accurately dose your blend, you need 5g of Milk thistle, turmeric, dandelion and Licorice root (red milligram scoop included), 30g of Glutamine (1/8 tsp scoop included), a digital milligram scale, and a mortar and pestle.

2. With your filler and your active ingredient appropriately mixed, can begin filling the capsules. Size 00 empty capsules will be needed, plus the Capsule Machine, and your mix. Load your empty capsules into the holes. The longer halves of the capsules go in the base; the shorter halves go in the lid.

3. Set the bottom of your capsule machine on its stand and set it on a plate or flat bowl to catch any powder that spilled. Then put some of your mixes onto it and use the accompanying scraper to fill the capsules.

4. Remove the base from the stand. You can now place the lid, of the capsule machine, containing the capsule tops on the base of the device. Securely, press down to join the

capsule ends together. The capsule machine base is on a rigid spring and should flatten with enough force.

5. You can now push down on the back of the lid to bring out your capsules.

Maintaining a Healthy Lifestyle Post-Treatment

Whether you are having type 1 or type 2 diabetes, it is a fact that all forms of diabetes are the presence of high amounts of sugar in your blood. This, therefore, implies that if you could own your own titrate or reduce your sugar intake, there would little or no work for your pancreas to do, and you would NEVER be labeled a DIABETIC. So I always advise that you focus your strategies of maintaining a "healthy you" to first principles. What do I mean? First principles for having a normal blood sugar will entail eating healthy, avoiding a sedentary lifestyle, enjoy herbal remedies, which have no drug reaction, and then the last but not the least, meditation and fasting.

According to Manuel I., who said in his testimony above "a lousy mixture of over drinking alcohol, eating fast foods and no exercising routinely " it is indeed true that 99% of diabetic cases are the result of multiple factors rather than a single causative agent. So you should not expect a single method that fixes all shortcomings neither should you expect damage of over twenty (20) years to be repaired in a month or less.

Before the commencement of herbal treatment to reverse your diabetes, it is relevant and instructive to bear in mind that our treatment program for both types of diabetes should be focused on diet improvement and lifestyle changes.

The Atkins Diet states that it's eating plan can prevent or improve severe health conditions, such as high blood pressure, and diabetes. Note that, almost any diet that helps you shed excess weight can reduce or even reverse risk factors for diabetes.

Low carb plus healthy fat meal or Ketogenic diet in addition to regular fasting at intervals is also highly recommended as a precursor to the suggested herbal treatment, for fast results.

The following steps must be collectively applied as a daily routine to maintain good health thus ensuring you never suffer a return of high blood sugar referred to as diabetes:

- Drastically reduce or cut out all the sugars and refined carbohydrates from your daily food intake.

- Keep up with your daily exercise routine. Add yoga in the evenings, before you go to bed.

- Stay active. Keep your mind positively engaged. This is very important for seniors.

- Walking around for 15-30 mins after meals and last but not the least;

- Fast at regular intervals. The appropriate method for doing this is explained in my book *"Meditation and Fasting Combined: A Powerful Healer."*

6.1 Foods to Avoid

Dried Fruit, Trans Fats, White Bread, Pasta and Rice, Fruit-Flavored Yogurt, Sweetened Breakfast Cereals, Sugar-Sweetened Beverages, Flavored Coffee Drinks, Honey, Agave Nectar and Maple Syrup.

Sugary beverages are the worst drink choice for someone with diabetes.

Herbal remedies for routine maintenance, Exercises, meditation and fasting techniques, and other diet programs will be extensively discussed in my new book *"After Reversing Diabetes: Herbal Remedies to Avoid Relapse."*

Achieving diabetes remission is not easy by any standard, and involves several disturbing lifestyle chances, but your hard work in reducing and maintaining an appropriate weight in line with your body mass index and also keeping blood sugar levels is just as essential now as upon entering remission. Many will struggle to accomplish the long-term reversal of type 2 diabetes. Though not easy, it is achievable.